MEDICARE DECODED

SHOCKING FACTS
to help you save money and
get the most from Medicare

RICK SOLOFSKY

SENIOR ADVOCATES PRESS

ISBN: 978-0-578-65535-2

Printed in the United States of America

Contents

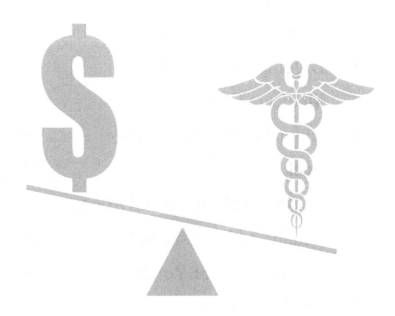

INTRODUCTION

I am a passionate man.

Most of us are passionate about something (at least I *hope* we are), be it sports or cars, learning or religion, or any number of other things that we use to help us focus our energies, talents, and intellects. Me, I have a passion for wrestling. Not that I do it much nowadays (I'm getting up there in years), but I've been able to stay engaged by officiating at over a hundred and sixty regional and national tournaments. I've directed my passion toward helping wrestlers become better men through my favorite sport. It's gratifying and humbling to look back on the lives that I've touched and to see how those competitors have grown into strong, productive, sometimes extraordinary people. In some small way, I've helped those men lead better lives. I feel pretty good about that.

My other passion is Medicare. Sounds weird, right? Okay, let me narrow it down a little: My other passion is *helping people better understand and utilize Medicare.* When I talk about Medicare I get so revved up that the ideas come a mile a minute. I can't express them quickly enough to make me happy, but I also can't slow down. I get excited about Medicare the way some people get excited about football or *Star Wars.* When I go to parties, people gather around me to listen. "Hey, everybody! Come over here! Rick's going to tell that Medicare story again!"

I know, it still sounds weird. I get it. But think about this: Unless you have an ongoing source of significant wealth, you can look forward to having a cozy relationship with Medicare in the future. Maybe you're having that relationship right now. I wouldn't be surprised: Approximately fifteen percent of the US population uses Medicare benefits. At the same time, almost sixteen percent of the US population is over sixty-five years old. In other words, *the overwhelming majority of the eligible population is using Medicare benefits*. And it gets even more serious: by 2027, a hundred and twenty million people, or over one third of the population, will be over age sixty-five. Sooner or later, Medicare is coming for all of us, but even if it's still far in your own future, who will take care of your aging parents? Look in the mirror. If you don't understand the ins and outs of Medicare now, you might find yourself footing the bill for a lot of caregiving that you never saw coming. I bet you'd be okay with dropping a couple of decimal places from your bank account, right?

I didn't think so. Very few of us have a solid, or even a rudimentary, understanding of how Medicare really works. It's a program that affects millions of people every single day. Your knowledge or ignorance of it will have serious life-and-death consequences and financial repercussions for you and your entire family. How much time and effort have you invested into exploring and mastering it? Probably not enough. Now would be a good time to get savvy. Maybe we should *all* be a little passionate about Medicare.

BUT WHY ON EARTH SHOULD I BELIEVE ANYTHING YOU SAY ABOUT MEDICARE?

Because I've spent the last three decades helping people maximize what Medicare has to offer. My company, Solofsky Financial Group, has administered plans for companies and individuals throughout the Mid-Atlantic for over thirty years. In short, I know what I'm talking about. My expertise is sought by attorneys, CEOs, brokers, business owners, and the media. And now, for the low, low price of this book, I'm going to share it with you. Between these covers I'll show you how to make sense of what can seem, at first, like an overwhelming topic. I'll also reveal some of Medicare's lesser known quirks and opportunities—essential things that many other guides leave out—that can make a big impact on your wallet and provide you with advantages that most people don't even know about. And, best of all, I promise you that this is the only Medicare book on the market that won't put you to sleep.

My work with Medicare, just like my work with wrestling, allows me to help people live better lives. And, just like my work with wrestling, I feel pretty good about it. As Mick Jagger said, "What a drag it is getting old" (and he should know). Aging is a challenge, but what I offer can make it just a little bit easier. I'd like to make it a little bit easier for *you*.

So grab a drink, put your phone on the table (screen side down), and settle in. Our story begins in the closing months of the Second World War. Time travel is difficult, but not for you. You only need to turn the page...

Chapter 1

THE BABY BOOM

As World War II wound down GIs began returning home to reunite with their families and the sweethearts they'd left behind. What they encountered when they landed back on American shores was a nation very different from the one they remembered from just a few short years ago. Gone was the decade-long funk of a worldwide depression and the existential threat of a world war. In their place was an overwhelming confidence in the future, a sense of optimism and pride born of a job well done. They had conquered enemies both economic and military, and now they would embark upon the unprecedented task of building a new, prosperous nation that would surpass anything the world had seen. Naturally, they did what any exuberant, forward-thinking population would do: They had lots of kids.

THE BABY BOOM

Most of us associate the Baby Boom with postwar euphoria, the era of Dwight Eisenhower, the birth of rock and roll, and young families making the most of newfound peace and prosperity. It was also the golden era of the growth of workplace benefits as employers began offering generous salaries, subsidized family healthcare, and an unspoken promise that a worker's loyalty and good performance would, in turn, earn the employer's loyalty and generosity.

In this bubble of security and contentment, with every reason to believe that our national good fortune would continue, it's little wonder that so many families took root and blossomed.

AMERICAN GENERATIONS OF THE 20TH AND 21ST CENTURIES

There is no consensus about exactly when generations begin and end (or how generations are named). This list reflects generally agreed-upon definitions.

The Greatest Generation
(Born 1901-1925)

This generation has the greatest name thanks to Tom Brokaw's 1998 bestseller *The Greatest Generation*. These are the people who brought us through the depression, saved democracy in World War Two, created un-precedented prosperity, passed landmark civil-rights legislation, and capped it off by putting a man on the Moon. The Greatest Generation indeed.

The Rock-n-Roll Generation
(Born 1926-1945)

They might have been *Leave it to Beaver* but they were also "Shake, Rattle, and Roll." They defined the modern teenager, but they also learned to conform and work within an established system, giving the 1950s their characteristic straight-laced reputation.

The Baby Boomers
(Born 1946-1964)

Here we are! This huge swell of the population became the GIs in Vietnam, the muddy campers of Woodstock, and the countercultural hippie kids of Haight-Ashbury.

They also ushered in a sense of social justice that continues to influence and inspire youth movements throughout the world.

Generation X
(Born 1965-1979)

The MTV Generation, the coffee achievers, the totally rad new wavers, Generation X refuses to be defined (hence the name), but if you're a part of it you get it. This group came of age during the AIDS epidemic and ushered in the post-Cold War world. Also sometimes called The Baby Busters because they were born during the steep decline of the birth rate following the Baby Boom.

Millennials
(Born 1980-2000)

If you're old you probably call this The Whiniest Generation. If you're young you think it's The Greatest Generation II. The jury's out, but one thing's for sure: This generation is indelibly shaped by the rise of the internet and the attacks of September 11th, 2001.

??????
(Born since 2001)

Some call it Generation Z, others call it the iGeneration, and it probably goes by one or two other names as well. The members of this generation are marked by a digital culture that infuses every aspect of their lives. Where will they lead us?

The Baby Boom began in 1946 when the US birthrate ballooned from 2,858,000 births the previous year to a staggering 3,411,000—by far the largest in the nation's history. While this is exactly when we would expect to start seeing the new children of recently returned veterans (World War II ended in 1945), these young families weren't the only ones being fruitful and multiplying. The one-two punch of depression and war had convinced many couples to postpone having children until better times were on the horizon. Now better times were here and the day had come to prepare the nursery for that little bundle of joy that for many years had only been a dream.

But the boom didn't end in the immediate postwar years. It actually expanded as families took advantage of the good vibes that continued from the late forties through the mid-sixties. The birth rate accelerated year after year, finally peaking in 1957 with over 4,300,000 births.

Opinions are divided about when the boom ended, but the US Census Bureau says that the ride was over in 1964. The birth rate wouldn't creep above the four-million mark again until 1989.

WHAT DOES THIS HAVE TO DO WITH MEDICARE?

Plenty. Medicare was launched in 1966 at the tail end of the Baby Boom during Lyndon Johnson's Administration (Harry and Bess Truman, the former president and first lady, were the first enrollees). At the time, approximately sixty percent of Americans aged sixty-five or older had health insurance, with many of the remainder unable to afford coverage due to their advanced age or pre-existing conditions. With the stroke of a pen, President Johnson changed the lives of millions of people.

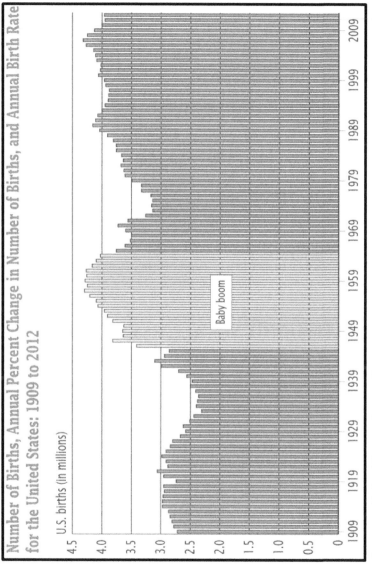

Number of Births, Annual Percent Change in Number of Births, and Annual Birth Rate for the United States: 1909 to 2012

U.S. births (in millions)

Baby boom

Courtesy United States Census Bureau

In 1966 a little under ten percent of the population was over sixty-five. In 2020, that number will be almost seventeen percent and, as average life expectancies continue to improve, the percentage of senior citizens will continue to increase. In other words, the ratio of older to younger Americans has shifted and there are fewer young, healthy Americans available to support an ever-aging group that relies upon Medicare for essential services.

WAIT: DON'T WE ALL PAY INTO OUR OWN PERSONAL MEDICARE FUNDS?

That's a common misconception. Younger workers pay taxes which are funneled into two trust funds that are used to provide Medicare services to senior citizens *today*. If you're earning and paying taxes, you are helping to pay for health care for *today's* seniors. Who will pay for yours?

We are getting older, we're enjoying longer lifespans, we have more age-related health problems (because we're living longer), and Medicare is paying for far more services and medications than it was initially intended to provide. It's a fabulously expensive program and the system is becoming top-heavy: As a percentage of the population, the older group that receives the benefits keeps getting larger while the younger group that pays for it all is shrinking. The number of workers per recipient has fallen from 4.6, when the program began in 1966, to approximately three in 2019, and this ratio is projected to continue falling for the foreseeable future. More old people means more Medicare recipients. Fewer workers means less money. It's a problem. A big one.

And it could be a big problem long before you're even eligible for Medicare benefits. The vast majority of people reading this book are approaching Medicare age because those are the people who buy books about Medicare. The ugly truth, though, is that this book needs to be read by people whose *parents* are approaching Medicare age. Remember, according to 1966 life expectancies, by the time you were eligible for Medicare your parents would likely have passed on. Nowadays, when you reach Medicare age, your parents are not only probably still alive, they're probably still running around like a couple of embarrassing teens. Times have changed!

We have reached a point where Medicare, which was designed to support one generation of seniors, is supporting *two* generations, along with all of the expensive health issues that develop as we grow older. There aren't enough people paying the bills to provide benefits to a population far larger than Medicare was designed to accommodate. What worked in 1966 doesn't work in the 21st century. The most obvious way to address the problem of an ever-increasing life expectancy is to increase the Medicare eligibility age from sixty-five to seventy, a change that will probably occur at some point, but it will literally take an act of Congress to get it done and that isn't likely to happen any time soon. In the meantime, we have to work with what we've got.

If your parents are enrolled in Medicare, or about to be, pay attention to how their plan is set up and the timing of their enrollments. You'll see explanations and warnings throughout this book to help you navigate expensive pitfalls. The stakes are high: A miscalculation or mis-understanding could jeopardize your parents' finances and well-being, and will also potentially eat into any inheritance that they plan to leave behind. And that impacts *you*.

WE'RE DOOMED!

Not quite. The demographic outlook isn't going to change anytime soon, but congress is unlikely to let the system fail—far too many people rely upon it. Nonetheless, in the absence of a major recalibration, there is the potential for higher contributions, curtailed services, and—brace yourself—government intervention. The good news is that there are things that you and I can do right here right and now that will ease the burden while delivering real benefits to you, to your employer, and to Uncle Sam. That's a win-win-win. Sound too good to be true? It's not. Read on!

Chapter 2

MEDICARE FROM A TO D

Like piloting a jet plane, Medicare can seem impenetrably complex to those who haven't had to deal with it, and jumping into the deep end of the Medicare pool can be like drinking from a firehose. Mixed metaphors aside, understanding Medicare is nowhere near as challenging as flying a 737. In fact, while it certainly requires some boning up, the whole program is a great deal simpler than most people realize. A little familiarity goes a long way; a short orientation will help you sort out what Medicare is and what it isn't, who is eligible for it and who is not, how to activate it when the time comes, and how to make sure that you understand how to make the various parts of Medicare work for you in the best possible way.

MEDICARE: BROUGHT TO YOU BY THE LETTERS A, B, C, AND D

The Medicare program is divided into four parts: Medicare Parts A, B, C, and D. Each part has a specific role to play and each one pays for different products and services (although Part C is a bit of an oddball—we'll get to that). Parts A and B are the original Medicare program that was inaugurated in 1966 during the Lyndon Johnson Administration. Parts C and D were added later. As with most government-administered programs, there is a lot of nitty-gritty granular detail that we could get into (and we will), but for now

I'm going to give you a brief general orientation on each part (all premiums, coverages, etc. are current as of 2019).

MEDICARE PART A

What Does Part A Do? Medicare Part A is often called the hospital insurance portion of Medicare, but that's a bit misleading. The term *hospital insurance* implies all-inclusive coverage, but that's not how this works. Part A pays for your hospital room and bed, but it does not pay for many of the services that you might receive while you're there. Part B takes care of those. So Part A and Part B split the responsibility for paying for your room, board, and nursing care (Part A), and most other medical services (Part B).

Who Is Eligible for Part A? Medicare, like slow driving, afternoon naps, and telling the kids to get off your lawn, is one of the hallmarks of growing old. Generally speaking, Medicare is available to every US citizen (or permanent legal resident of at least five continuous years) who also meets at least one of the following criteria:

Age sixty-five and Eligible for Social Security: Most people will automatically be enrolled in Medicare Part A when they turn sixty-five and become eligible for Social Security benefits.

Permanently Disabled and Collecting Disability Benefits for at Least Two Years: You will automatically be enrolled after receiving twenty-four months of benefits from Social Security or the Railroad Retirement Board.

Have Amyotrophic Lateral Sclerosis (ALS, or Lou Gehrig's Disease): You will automatically be enrolled the month that your benefits begin.

Have End-Stage Renal Disease (ESRD): If you require a kidney transplant or dialysis treatment, you are eligible for Medicare benefits. Unlike the previous scenarios, however, enrollment is not automatic. You must take the initiative to enroll.

What Does Part A Cover? In general, Part A covers...

- A semiprivate room, or a private room if medically necessary, in acute care, critical access, long-term care, inpatient rehab, and psychiatric hospitals, with a per-admission deductible of $1,364.00 in 2019
- Regular, facility-based nursing care as long as custodial care (meaning non-medical services ordinarily provided by nurse's aides) isn't the only care required.
- Meals, even if specially prepared to meet medical requirements
- Limited home-health services, to include part-time skilled nursing care, social services, various rehabilitative therapies, and durable medical equipment when ordered by a physician

Nursing-home care for inpatient admissions of three or more days

- Hospice care for terminally ill patients with an estimated six months or less to live.

What Does Part A NOT Cover? In general, Part A does not cover...

- Private hospital rooms unless medically necessary
- Private nurses
- Personal items and hospital add-ons, like cable TV fees.

How Much Does Part A Cost? If you or your spouse has paid Medicare taxes for at least forty quarters (that's ten years for you math whizzes) there is no premium for Part A. If you (or your spouse) have been gainfully employed for most of your adult life, then you have probably paid the necessary taxes for premium-free Part A participation. However, if you have paid Medicare taxes for *less than* thirty quarters (7 ½ years), or have NEVER paid them at all, Part A will cost you $437.00 per month. If you paid Medicare taxes for thirty to thirty-nine quarters (7 ½ to 9 ¾ years), it will cost you $240.00 per month (all as of 2019).

MEDICARE PART B

What Does Part B Do? Medicare Part B covers most medical services that are not already covered by Medicare Part A (which is to say *most* medical services). Part B pays for 80% of eligible services after a $185.00 (in 2019) annual deductible (which is why Medicare supplement plans, which help to pick up the slack left by Part B's coverage, are popular).

Who Is Eligible for Part B? Everyone who is eligible for Part A is also eligible for Part B, but enrollment is not automatic and a monthly premium is required. It is crucial that you enroll in Part B at the right time or you will risk a permanent financial penalty—ten percent additional premium, for the duration of your enrollment, for every twelve-month period that you could have enrolled but didn't—and gaps in coverage while you wait for the open enrollment period to come around (see Chapter Five, "Annual Open Enrollment," for more). Neither of these is an attractive situation, but there is an exception if you are still employed and covered by your employer's health plan. See Chapter Four, "Medicare Secondary Payer," for details.

What Does Part B Cover? In general, Part B covers...

- Medically necessary services (including surgeries)

- Equipment, including durable medical equipment, that is required to diagnose and treat medical conditions
- Preventive services intended to identify and prevent health problems and conditions
- Ambulance services when private transportation may be harmful to the patient
- Physician-administered drugs
- Outpatient physical and speech therapies.

What Does Part B NOT Cover? In general, Part B does not cover...

- Vaccinations and immunizations
- Elective medical treatments
- Long-term care
- Alternative medicine (with a partial exception for chiropractic treatments)
- Dental work
- Eye and ear exams; glasses and hearing aids

- Routine podiatry
- Prescription drugs taken at home, and over-the-counter medications.

How Much Does Part B Cost? As of 2019, Medicare Part B requires a monthly premium that begins at $135.50 for those with annual incomes of $85,000 or less ($170,000 or less for couples), increasing incrementally to $460.50 for those with annual incomes of $500,000 or more ($750,000 or more for couples).

MEDICARE PART D

Wait, What Happened to Medicare Part C? As I said at the beginning of this chapter, Part C is an oddball and it'll be easier to explain it after we talk about Part D. So let's talk about Part D!

What Does Part D Do? Medicare Part D is, simply put, Medicare's prescription plan, but unlike Parts A and B, which are administered by the Federal Government, Part D is administered by private insurers and there are a number of plans available.

Who Is Eligible for Part D? Anyone who is eligible for Part A but, like Part B, Part D requires enrollment. It isn't automatic. Also, while each plan covers a wide selection of drugs, none of them cover *all* the drugs, and you can only pick one plan. If you're the type who agonizes over what to order from the lunch menu at Subway, you're going to have a ball with Medicare Part D. Additionally, if you don't sign up during your first open enrollment period (October 15th through December 7th) you will pay a one-percent penalty for every month that you delayed enrollment. The decisions that you have to make with Part D give you all of the ingredients for a fun afternoon at the kitchen table trying to sort out the pros and cons.

What Does Part D Cover? Like most con-ventional prescription plans, Part D helps pay for medications prescribed by a physician, although there is a coverage gap (see *How Much Does Part D Cost?* below).

What Does Part D NOT Cover? Part D does not help pay for over-the-counter medications, certain sedatives, tranquilizers, and weight-loss drugs, Viagra, Cialis (unless prescribed as a blood thinner for a medically diagnosed issue), or (big surprise here) any illegal pharmaceuticals.

How Much Does Part D Cost? Like most non-Medicare prescription plans, Part D generally requires a monthly premium, but exactly how much that is depends upon the plan that you select. Expect to spend less than—and maybe *significantly* less than—$100 a month. In fact, most plans cost around twenty to thirty dollars a month. Also, like most other private prescription plans, Part D plans often require copays when picking up drugs at the pharmacy. In addition to these costs, Part D has a unique blackout period, or coverage gap, that causes a great deal of consternation among participants. Simply put, Part D puts a cap on how much you and your carrier will pay annually to cover your prescription medications. In 2019 that annual cap is $3,820.00. When that limit is reached, your out-of-pocket expenses may increase dramatically until your annual costs reach $5,100.00. After *that* your plan will pay ninety-five percent of all pharmacy expenses until the end of the year when the whole cycle begins anew (for more information, see Chapter Three, "Digging Into Part D").

MEDICARE PART C

What Does Part C Do? Medicare Part C's name causes a little confusion, and no wonder: Medicare Parts A, B, and D are all separate components that complement one another and, when assembled together, create a fairly comprehensive health-insurance program. Part C is completely different. Often called *Medicare Advantage Plans,* Part C plans are offered by private insurers through health maintenance organizations (HMOs) or preferred provider organizations (PPOs) as an alternative to the Medicare plans offered by the government.

The Federal Government has partnered with private insurers to make Part C plans as attractive as possible in an effort to move people off of traditional Medicare plans. Why would they go to all of the trouble to design an awesome health-care plan and then try to tempt people away with this private alternative? Because in 2003, the George W. Bush Administration saw a tsunami on the horizon: millions of Baby Boomers were about to reach Medicare age while their parents, already enrolled, were still healthy and showed no signs of dying off! This was an unprecedented situation and the scope of the oncoming influx threatened to swamp the system. They came up with an interesting solution: In exchange for allowing private insurers to collect monthly Medicare premiums from the public, along with a monthly per-member payment provided by the government, private companies assumed the risk of insuring millions of people, relieving the government of that responsibility. Think about that: The government has a load off its back; private insurers collect premiums and subsidies; and members, in most cases, receive more robust options. Everyone wins.

Who Is Eligible for Part C? Because Part C plans are wholly private, the eligibility is determined by each individual insurer. If you see a plan that you like, check the requirements to see if you qualify.

What Does Part C Cover? By law, Part C plans must cover everything that Parts A and B cover (and they often include prescription plans that replace Part D as well). In addition to duplicating traditional Medicare coverage, Part C plans may also cover additional services such as vision, dental, and hearing exams.

What Does Part C NOT Cover? That depends upon the insurer. Part C plans are only *required* to provide coverage identical to traditional Medicare.

How Much Does Part C Cost? Once again, that depends upon the insurer, but you can count on monthly premiums, and probably copays and any other costs that accompany most health-insurance plans. When considering a Medicare Advantage Plan, carefully weigh the benefits of a private plan against the associated costs to determine if it's right for you. And bear in mind that, every year, your provider will have an opportunity to raise premiums or drop out of the program altogether.

And be careful: In their enthusiasm to entice people to join Part C, no-premium plans (which are exactly what they sound like) and Private Fee for Service, or PFFS, plans (which often allow more freedom to select caregivers) are available that seem almost too good to be true. The catch is that they have *much* higher hospitalization daily copays, up to $300 a day in 2019. When you buy one of these plans, you're rolling the dice: You may save a lot of money in the long run, but a few days in the hospital might wipe out your bank account.

AND THEN THERE'S MEDIGAP

Just to be clear, Medigap plans are NOT a part of Medicare. Like Part C plans, Medigap plans are offered by private companies; unlike Part C plans, Medigap is not designed to be an alternative to other Medicare plans. On the contrary, Medigap plans are designed to supplement existing Medicare plans and pay for things that your basic insurance doesn't cover. Medigap plans are, for the most part, outside of the scope of this book (check with providers to see what's available), but here's a quick rundown of what they're all about:

Who is Eligible for Medigap Plans? Anyone who is enrolled in Part A and Part B is eligible to buy a Medigap plan. Medigap plans are NOT available to those enrolled in Medicare Advantage (Part C) plans.

What do Medigap Plans Cover? Medigap plans attempt to plug some of the coverage holes in Parts A and B, things like co-pays, deductibles, hospital and skilled-nursing facility costs after your Medicare coverage has run out, and health-care coverage outside of the United States.

What do Medigap Plans NOT Cover? Medigap does not cover eyeglasses, hearing aids, private nurses, and prescription drugs (although some older plans do have prescription components).

How Much do Medigap Plans Cost? Medigap plans are offered by private insurers and their premiums may vary widely. Shop around. If you are considering a Medicare Advantage (Part C) plan, compare Part C's benefits and costs to what your insurer's Medigap plan would offer when combined with Parts A and B. Remember, Medigap cannot be combined with Medicare Advantage, so weigh the pros and cons and make the choice that's right for you.

CONGRATULATIONS! YOU NOW KNOW MORE ABOUT MEDICARE THAN EIGHTY-FIVE PERCENT OF THE US POPULATION

I can't actually verify that statistic, but this much is true: If you read, understand, and remember this summary of the four parts of Medicare (and Medigap) you will have gained a better comprehension of our nation's massive health-care program than most of your peers. You're already ahead of the game. Now it's time to put on your greasy coveralls and prepare to get your hands dirty. We're going to raise the hood on this beast and poke around in the engine to discover how you can optimize Medicare to deliver the best possible service with the smallest impact on your checkbook.

Chapter 3

DIGGING INTO PART D

Medicare didn't always have a prescription plan. And prescriptions didn't always cost as much as Hawaiian vacations. As drug costs skyrocketed, and ordinary Americans found themselves unable to afford the medications that they desperately needed, the wheels of government slowly started to turn. After an aborted attempt by the Clinton administration, George W. Bush's administration overcame legislative challenges to pass a Medicare Part D bill into law, finally granting some relief to millions of financially strapped senior citizens.

As great as that was (and is) it came with a weird coverage gap that came to be known as the *donut hole,* one of the most hated and feared aspects of Medicare.

THE DREADED DONUT HOLE

There's good news! But before we jump into that, we need to talk a little more about this phenomenon. The donut hole has such a fearsome reputation that Medicare newbies will probably keep hearing about worst-case scenarios from uninformed sources even as this issue changes and evolves. That's why you need to know the hole truth (see what I did there?).

When Medicare Part D was born in 2003 it included the following provision: Medicare Part D covered annual prescription costs (exclusive of copays) until $3,820 had been expended. At that point, the beneficiary (you) had to pay one hundred percent of prescription costs until $5,100 had been paid. That's $5,100 out of your own pocket. Afterward, Part D would cover ninety-five percent of prescription costs for the rest of the year (this was known as *catastrophic coverage*).

With drug prices soaring ever higher, participants were overspending their $3,820 caps with alarming regularity, and the threat (and all too often the reality) of having to shell out as much as $5,100 every single year caused much wailing and gnashing of teeth among the senior population and its caregivers (who increasingly had to pony up with their own money to help their aging parents and grandparents afford their medications).

SWEET RELIEF

And here's the good news that I told you about: Thankfully, the government heard our anguished pleas and started making changes to Part D to reduce the hardships caused by the infamous donut hole. Instead of requiring participants to pay the full amount of their prescription medications after falling into the coverage gap, Uncle Sam started paying a portion, gradually increasing it over time.

DON'T SKIP THIS PART!
THE THREE PHASES OF MEDICARE PART D

The rationale and calculations that form the basis for the way that Medicare Part D works are locked in a vault in Area 51 along with other enduring mysteries of the last half-century (and this is a JOKE; please don't go to Area 51 to "get a look at" the secret Medicare books, and if you do, please don't mention my name). **This is one of the most misunderstood aspects of Medicare and one that can result in nasty financial surprises if you aren't paying attention.**

Here's how the program works in 2019: Medicare Part D plans are private prescription plans offered by private insurers with the participation of, and supervised by, the federal government. As with any private insurance, you pay a monthly premium (usually between thirty-five and thirty-seven dollars), and when you purchase prescription drugs you may be responsible for a copay that is set by your insurer (check with them). Part D is an annual plan (meaning that everything resets to zero on January 1st of every calendar year regardless of the month of your enrollment). The coverage is divided into three distinct phases.

PHASE 1: Initial Coverage Period: $3,820

When you enroll in Medicare Part D, you are automatically in Phase 1 and you'll stay there until your pharmacist's average wholesale cost (the amount that your pharmacist pays for your drugs) AND your copays (the amount that you spend at the cash register) reach or exceed $3,820 (at which point you move into Phase 2). $3,820 seems like a lot of money, but it can add up quickly, especially if you can't use generics. Here are a couple of examples of how Phase 1 works:

Phase 1, Example 1

Your doctor prescribes you five drugs which you must purchase on a monthly basis. Generics are available. On January 1st, you buy the five *generic* prescription drugs that your doctor prescribed and you owe $5.00 copay for each one: **5 generic drugs x $5.00 copay = $25.00 copay (paid by *you*) per month.**

Your parmacist's average wholesale cost for each of these five generic drugs is $3.00. **5 generic drugs x $3.00 average wholesale cost = $15.00 average wholesale cost (paid by *your pharmacist*) per month.**

$25.00 in copays (paid by you) + $15.00 average wholesale cost (paid by your pharmacist) = $40.00 *total* monthly payment.

You have to take these drugs every month, therefore: **$40.00 total monthly payment x 12 months = *$480.00 total annual payment.***

In this case, $3,780 is plenty of coverage. No big deal, right? Sure. But what if generics aren't available? What if you have to take an expensive brand-name prescription like Lipitor? Suddenly the numbers may not look so good. Here's an example.

Phase 1, Example 2

On January 1st, you buy the five *brand-name* prescription drugs that your doctor prescribed and you owe $50.00 copay for each one: **5 brand-name drugs x $50.00 copay = $250.00 copay (paid by *you*) per month.**

Your parmacist's average wholesale cost for each of these five generic drugs is $200.00. **5 name-brand drugs x $200.00 average wholesale cost = $1,000.00 average wholesale cost (paid by *your pharmacist*) per month.**

$250.00 in copays (paid by you) + $1,000.00 average wholesale cost (paid by your pharmacist) = $1,250.00 *total* monthly payment.

You have to take these drugs every month, therefore: **$1,250.00 total monthly payment x 12 months = *$15,000.00 total annual payment.***

In fact, you will nearly reach the $3,820 threshold (after which you enter Phase 2) by the end of March. Once you cross that threshold you will enter Phase 2: the *coverage gap,* AKA the dreaded Medicare *donut hole.*

PHASE 2: Coverage gap

While you'll still owe a portion of the costs, things are a heck of a lot better than they used to be: While in the coverage gap, you used to be responsible for one hundred percent of the cost of any prescription drugs until you had paid $5,100—a financial disaster for many older Americans. But things have changed. In 2019, Instead of paying one hundred percent of the *retail price* (not the *average wholesale* cost that your pharmacist paid in Phase 1) of a prescription drug, you are now responsible for only thirty-seven percent of the retail price until you have paid $5,100 out of pocket (and bear in mind the fact that, if we're talking about expensive name-brand prescriptions, even thirty-seven percent of the retail price could be an exorbitant sum).

As of 2020, you will only be responsible for twenty-five percent of the retail price of your prescription drugs while in Phase 2 until you have paid $5,100 out of pocket (the $5,100 total expense that you are responsible for hasn't changed). More good news: As of 2020, while you're in the donut hole, every time you buy a medication and pay twenty-five percent of the retail price, *ninety-five percent of the retail price will be credited toward the $5,100 coverage gap.* So if your drug retails for $100, while you're in the coverage gap you will pay $25, but $95 will go against the $5,100 that must be paid in order to close the donut hole and move on to Phase 3. This helps you move out of the coverage gap far more rapidly than if the system only counted the money that you actually spent. Pretty cool, huh?

After you have fulfilled the $5,100 obligation you will move into Phase 3 for the remainder of the calendar year.

Phase 3: Catastrophic coverage

Phase 3, called *catastrophic coverage,* is the best phase of all (and the fact that so many of us find ourselves reaching a phase that's called *catastrophic coverage* tells you something about how much the cost of prescription drugs has skyrocketed in recent years. It's no longer catastrophic; it's normal). After you have surpassed your $5,100 obligation in Phase 2, Medicare Part D will cover your prescription costs to the tune of ninety-five percent. You pay five percent of the cost of your prescriptions for the rest of the year. That's a great deal, but you have to jump through the hoops of Phase 1 and Phase 2 to get there. After that, the cycle begins again. And that's Medicare Part D!

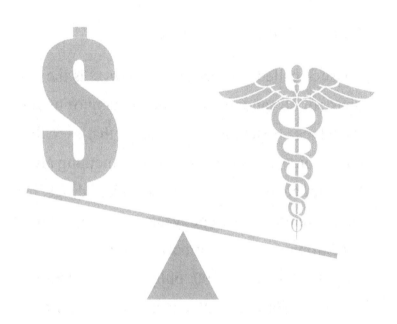

Chapter 4

MEDICARE SECONDARY PAYER

Now that we have the basics out of the way it's time to poke around in some of the lesser known areas of Medicare. This is important stuff: The nooks and crannies are where you'll find some of the best ways to make Medicare work for you in the best possible way for the least amount of money. Pay attention, because some of what you'll read here you won't find covered in depth in most other publications.

One of the most poorly understood issues is *Medicare Secondary Payer*. As our population ages and health care improves, we are, on average, spending a longer time in the workforce. Many of us are still gainfully employed on their sixty-fifth birthdays, when we become eligible for Medicare, and we may still be working for several years thereafter. If this describes your situation, and if your employer offers health-care coverage, there are some vitally important things that you can't afford not to know.

SORT YOURSELF OUT

First of all, if you are employed at age sixty-five *and* your employer offers health-care insurance, determine which of these three categories you're in:

- **Category 1:** Your company has nineteen or fewer employees

- **Category 2:** Your company has twenty or more employees
- **Category 3:** Your company has between two and ninety-nine employees and your spouse has been approved for Social Security disability. If this is you, listen up: This one is a doozy!

One more thing: When determining which of the above describes your situation, remember the following: The number of employees includes part-timers, seasonal, and union employees who *may not even be eligible for healthcare benefits.* Why? I have no idea, and they didn't consult me when they made the rules (unfortunately). My advice: Don't think about it too hard; you'll give yourself a headache. Just follow the rules. If you don't, the ache will be in your bank account instead of in your head.

If you are in Category 1 (Your company offers a health plan and has nineteen or fewer

employees): In groups with nineteen or fewer employees Medicare is the *primary payer.* This means that Medicare is the *primary plan of insurance coverage,* and the group coverage, which is provided by your employer, is the *secondary plan of coverage.* In this scenario, Medicare will pay benefits until the benefits are exhausted, and then your employer's plan will take over and continue to pay subject to its own rules and conditions.

Many who are still working at age sixty-five for a company that offers a health-care plan neglect to enroll in Medicare Part B (remember, most people are *automatically* enrolled in Part A when they turn sixty-five and become eligible for Social Security benefits). After all, why should they enroll in Part B? Their employer offers coverage, so they can always enroll later.

Here's why putting it off is a bad idea: Most group insurance carriers have a steadfast rule that if you work for a group of nineteen or fewer employees, and you do not apply for Medicare Part B (opting instead to stay covered exclusively by the group plan), and then have a claim, the group insurance carrier reserves the right to pay only twenty percent of the claim. Why? *Most group plans assume that you will enroll in Medicare Part B when you turn sixty-five.* Therefore, it's very much in your best interest to enroll in Medicare Part B.

Should you also enroll in a *Medicare Supplement,* or *Medigap,* plan? Absolutely. I know what you're thinking: "If Part B covers eighty percent of all claims (after a small deductible), why should I spend my money on a Medigap plan? I'll just pay the remaining twenty percent myself." Excellent. Maybe you will save some money. Unless you have a $200,000 surgical procedure (which, as you age, is increasingly likely to happen). Suddenly, that twenty percent that you owe is a $40,000 hospital bill. Can your checking account handle that? If it can, put this book down and hire a personal Medicare expert (like me) to figure all of this stuff out for you. If it can't, then you need to purchase a Medigap plan to fill in that twenty percent that the Medicare plans leave unfilled.

IN SHORT: If you are in category 1, enroll in Part B and get a Medigap plan and get off of your group plan. You employer will love you for it!

If you are in Category 2 (Your company offers a health plan and has twenty or more employees): The exact opposite of Category 1 is now the rule: For groups with twenty or more employees, Medicare is the *secondary payer* to the employer's group plan. This means that Medicare is the *secondary plan of insurance coverage,* and the group coverage, which is provided by your employer, is the *primary plan of coverage.* If you work for a company that employs twenty or more people (and remember that this number includes part-timers, seasonal employees, etc.), you do *not* have to apply for Medicare. This is where the trouble begins.

Your parents, your grandparents, your aunts and uncles, and your family friends probably all applied for Medicare when they turned age sixty-five, and you know this because that's the kind of thing that old people like to talk about and you overheard them. So if that's what the old people did, why should things be any different for me? *Here's* why: When people turned sixty-five in the late sixties, the seventies, and the early eighties, most of them were already retired or were retiring soon. In the past, applying for Medicare at age sixty-five was the norm. It was the way of life! But our average life expectancy is increasing and we're putting in more years at work. More years at work potentially means more years covered by an employer's health-care plan which, in turn, means that you can put off enrolling in Medicare, without fear of penalty, until you retire. This rule applies for as long as you're working and covered by your employer's program, even if you're ninety years old.

However, once you do retire, the clock starts ticking: You have three months from the date of your retirement to enroll in Medicare. If you fail to do so, the normal restrictions and penalties will kick in: You won't be able to apply for Medicare until the following January 1st to March 31st, your coverage won't begin until July 1st and you'll receive a permanent ten percent penalty on your premium for not applying on time. You'll pay a ten percent penalty for the rest of your life and you'll risk being without coverage for several months. The moral of the story: Enroll within three months of retirement and avoid the hassle.

If you are in Category 3 (Your company has between two and ninety-nine employees and your spouse has been approved for Social Security disability): Brace yourself: If you are in this situation an entirely different set of rules applies. If you work for company with between two and ninety-nine employees, *and* you are covered on your employer's plan, *and* you are covering your spouse, *and* your spouse is accepted for Social Security Disability, Medicare becomes your **primary payer** and your spouse MUST apply for Medicare Part A and Part B within twenty-four months of being approved for Social Security Disability.

However (you knew this was coming), if you work for a company that has one hundred employees or more, and you are covered on your employer's plan, *and* you are covering your spouse, *and* your spouse is accepted for Social Security Disability, your spouse does NOT have to apply for Medicare Part A and Part B. In this situation, Medicare is the **secondary payer** to the group coverage. In fact, if your spouse applied for Medicare Parts A and B in this situation, and you are paying for Medicare Part B, then he or she may be entitled to a refund of every Medicare premium that was paid.

SAVING THE BEST FOR LAST

Here's a little-known opportunity that very few people are aware of, one that could save employers hundreds of thousands of dollars, and provide better care options for employees: If an employer has employees on their group plan who are aged sixty-five and up their group premiums have probably shot through the roof. That's what happens when you have senior citizens in your group plan! However, if the employee requests to be removed from the group plan, *even if they continue to work,* they can potentially save their employer something in the neighborhood of ten to fifteen thousand dollars a year. And if another senior employee comes off the plan that's *another* ten to fifteen thousand saved. I know what you're thinking: "That's great for my boss, but what's in it for *me?*" Easy. Medicare, along with a supplement plan, is a much stronger plan of coverage than most employer-provided group insurance plan. Unless your company offers a Rolls Royce insurance plan (and very few do) you're better off on Medicare. This is huge! And it's completely overlooked by hundreds of thousands of business owners and millions of employees. If you're over sixty-five and on a company health-care plan, take a close look at it, see how it compares to what Medicare offers, see how the premiums stack up, and make the choice that's best for you. Then pat yourself on the back for discovering that you have options that most of your friends and coworkers never knew existed.

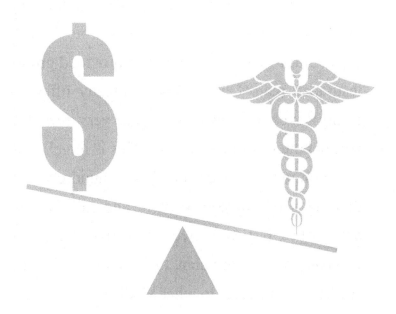

Chapter 5

ANNUAL OPEN ENROLLMENT

I know it's difficult to believe that there could be anything *confusing* **about Medicare** (that's a joke!), but one thing that continually befuddles people is *Medicare annual open enrollment.* It's a good thing I'm here to clear things up. Let's have a look...

THAT'S WHY THEY CALL IT *ANNUAL*...

Once you are enrolled in Medicare you will have an opportunity, once a year, to switch from a traditional government-administered Medicare plan (Part A and Part B) to a private Medicare Advantage plan (Part C) or vice versa. You can also switch your Part D plan (which is always privately administered) to a different Part D plan. If you neglected to enroll in Part D to begin with, the annual open enrollment period is your chance, although a late-enrollment fee may apply.

Mark your calendar: Open enrollment is generally from October 15th through December 7th every year (but double-check: As with everything else in this book, there's no guarantee that the powers-that-be won't make changes in the future). During that period you can do the following:

- If you're enrolled in traditional Medicare (Part A and Part B) you can switch to a private Medicare Advantage plan (Part C).

- If you're enrolled in a private Medicare Advantage Plan (Part C) you can switch to a traditional Medicare plan (Part A and Part B).

- If you're enrolled in a private Medicare Advantage plan (Part C) you can switch to a different Medicare Advantage plan.

- You can switch from one Part D plan to another Part D plan.

- If you aren't enrolled in Part D you may do so but a late-enrollment fee may apply.

WHAT IF I DON'T WANT TO CHANGE ANYTHING?

Then you don't have to change anything! Just sit back and relax; your existing coverage will continue.

WHAT IF I NEVER ENROLLED IN MEDICARE TO BEGIN WITH?

If, for whatever reason, you weren't enrolled in Medicare upon your sixty-fifth birthday, you may do so during the annual open enrollment period, but you may face a penalty of ten percent additional premium for every twelve-month period in which you were eligible for Medicare but weren't enrolled. See Chapter Four, "Medicare Secondary Payer," for more information about how work-provided health care may affect late enrollment.

WHAT IF I WANT TO MAKE CHANGES AND I CAN'T WAIT FOR THE ANNUAL OPEN ENROLLMENT PERIOD?

You have an additional opportunity to make some changes from January 1st through March

31st, but there are more restrictions and more penalties.

- If you're enrolled in a private Medicare Advantage Plan (Part C) you can switch to a traditional Medicare plan (Part A and Part B) and buy a Part D prescription plan. You may NOT switch from traditional Medicare to Medicare Advantage or make changes to an existing Part D plan.

- If, for whatever reason, you weren't enrolled in Medicare upon your sixty-fifth birthday, you may do so, but you may face a penalty of ten percent additional premium for every twelve-month period in which you were eligible for Medicare but weren't enrolled, AND your new Medicare coverage will not take effect until July 1st of the current year, **potentially leaving you without health coverage for as long as six months.**

This January-to-March period provides a little bit of a safety valve and some leeway in case things don't go as planned during the normal annual open enrollment period. The best way to make sure that things *do* go as planned is to plan. The January-to-March extension is there if you need it, but it's always best to make your changes during the annual open enrollment period.

WAIT: WHAT IF I WANT TO ENROLL IN OR MAKE CHANGES TO A MEDIGAP PLAN?

Go right ahead! Medigap (Medicare supplement) plans are offered by private insurers and are NOT governed by Medicare's open-enrollment rules. This does not mean that the company that provides your Medigap plan may not have its own set of enrollment rules; on the contrary, it very well might. Check with them, but don't worry about what Medicare might think.

Whatever you want to do with your Medigap coverage is okay with Medicare.

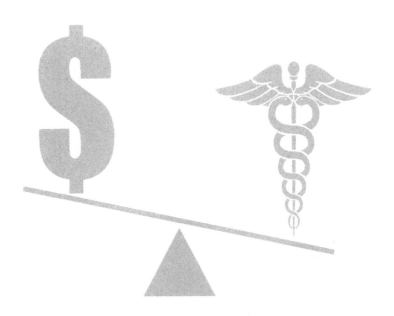

Chapter 6

BACK TO WORK

Mary suffered an accident that left her disabled and unable to work. She is under sixty-five, but because she is receiving Social Security disability income payments she was able to enroll in Medicare as a disabled person (see Chapter Four, "Medicare Secondary Payer," for more information about SSDI and Medicare).

After a few years, even though she is still defined as disabled, Mary feels that she is able to—and wants to—return to work. She contacts her employer and gets back on the payroll. She notifies Medicare of her change of status and is surprised to learn that she can continue to keep her Medicare benefits for *eight and a half years,* even though she is under sixty-five and wouldn't otherwise be eligible for Medicare benefits. Medicare Part A is premium-free and Mary continues to pay for Part B, as usual. This certainly makes things easier for Mary.

Why is she allowed to keep her Medicare benefits for so long? One reason is to ensure that Mary—and everyone else using Medicare while on disability—is properly taken care of. Another is that Medicare has determined that when someone who is receiving Social Security disability income goes back to work, that person is likely to receive disability income again within a few years of returning to the workplace. In other words, if your condition is bad enough to make you unemployable, it will probably make you unemployable again, and it's easier to keep you on the program than it is to remove you and reinstate you later (They're betting that you'll relapse, so if you need a little more incentive to maintain your health, there it is).

What if Mary, after returning to work, decides to re-enroll in the private health-care coverage provided by her employer? In this case, she can still keep her Medicare coverage for the full eight and a half years, under the same rules that we discussed in Chapter Four ("Medicare Secondary Payer"):

- If your employer has nineteen or fewer employees (including part-time and seasonal) Medicare is the *primary payer* and your employer's plan is the *secondary payer*. Medicare will pay benefits until the benefits are exhausted, and then your employer's plan will take over and continue to pay subject to its own rules and conditions.

- If your employer has twenty or more employees (including part-time and seasonal) Medicare is the *secondary payer* and your employer's plan is the *primary payer*. Your employer's plan will pay first subject to its own terms and conditions, and Medicare will pick up the slack when you exceed your employer's coverage.

WHAT HAPPENS AFTER EIGHT AND A HALF YEARS?

After eight and a half years, everything proceeds as it normally would. If Mary is still under sixty-five she'll have to do without Medicare. When she does turn sixty-five she can enroll in Medicare just like every other sixty-five-year-old. If she goes back on Social Security disability she could begin that process again as well.

Here's something to remember about Medicare's continuing coverage when returning to work after disability: In a program that often seems cold and heartless (as government systems often do), it's a reminder that, at its core, Medicare was designed to take care of us as we enter the last quarters of our lives, when we are often most vulnerable of most in need of help. It's not a bad thing to keep in mind.

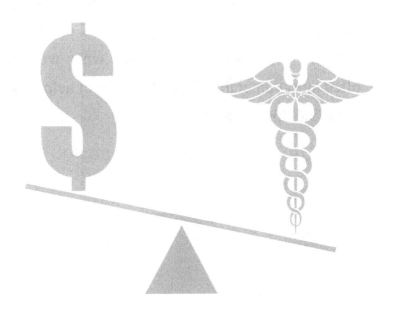

Chapter 7

RETIREMENT STUFF AND COBRA

What if I stay on my employer's plan, retire well past my sixty-fifth birthday, and *then* enroll in Medicare Part B? You can! I know what you're thinking: "But I'll owe that ten percent per year penalty that you talked about in Chapter Two (ten percent additional premium, for the duration of your enrollment, for every twelve-month period that you could have enrolled but didn't), right?"

Wrong! This is the exception that I mentioned in that same paragraph way back in Chapter Two. If you are covered by your employer's health-care plan past the age of sixty-five, you retire, and then enroll in Medicare Parts B and D (because you should already be enrolled in Part A) you will incur NO penalty as long as you enroll within three months. This three-month window is known as a *special enrollment period,* or SEP, and it's vital that you enroll within this period If you don't, your enrollment clock will reset to the date of your retirement or the date that your employer-supplied health insurance ended (whichever is later) and you will risk paying late-enrollment penalties for the entirety of your Medicare Parts B and D enrollment. Bear in mind that all of this also applies if the coverage belongs to your spouse.

IMPORTANT: When you disenroll from your employer's health-care plan, your employer's health-insurance provider will mail you a *creditable coverage letter*. This is an essential document and, like most official government documents, it still comes in the old-fashioned snail mail, so if you're in the habit of pitching anything that strikes you as junk, be careful. The creditable coverage letter is what tells Medicare that they cannot assess late-enrollment penalties against you as long as you enroll during the special enrollment period. It's the smoking gun that gets you off the hook. Don't lose it.

What if I'm bored with retirement, relapse, and go back to work? If you're the type who just can't stay away from the workplace, never fear: You can cancel Parts B and D and go back on your employer's plan. Once again you'll be like any other post-sixty-five-year-old on the job, with employer-provided health care and Medicare Part A running in tandem with one another. When you get tired of the office politics and retire again, you'll do the same thing that you did before: disenroll from your employer's plan, get a creditable coverage letter, and re-enroll in Medicare Parts B and D within an eight month special enrollment period. I know it seems like it should be more complicated than that, but it isn't. It's simple, it's straightforward, and it makes perfect sense. Who says the government never makes anything easy?

THE COBRA CONUNDRUM

If you're on a COBRA plan and under sixty-five, great. You're on COBRA; end of story.

If you're on COBRA when you turn sixty-five, you have to enroll in all parts of Medicare during your initial enrollment period just as you normally would if you were already retired. Failure to enroll in Medicare will result in the same lifelong penalties that would be applied to any retired person over sixty-five who misses their enrollment deadline. In other words, being on COBRA does not give you the same flexibility as being on an employer-sponsored plan.

If you are on COBRA when you enroll in Medicare, COBRA will become the *secondary* payer and Medicare will become the *primary* payer, just like being on an employer-sponsored plan at a company with less than twenty employees. If you are under sixty-five and on COBRA, then when you turn sixty-five you must enroll in Medicare Parts A and B during your Initial Enrollment Period. You are welcome to keep your COBRA plan and let it pay secondary instead of a Medigap plan, but remember that you must enroll in both Part A and Part B when you turn sixty-five.

If you choose to buy a COBRA plan upon retirement at or after your sixty-fifth birthday, then you must enroll in Medicare Parts B and D no later than your eighth month on the COBRA plan. Once again, failure to do so will result in lifetime penalties for late enrollment and a significant lapse in coverage while you wait for the open-enrollment period to come around. I call this *The Gotcha Rule,* and the penalties and coverage lapses can put you in a world of hurt (if you find yourself faced with the Gotcha Rule, check out Chapter Nine, "The Fountain of Youth," for a possible solution). Don't forget! Put a note on the refrigerator. Neglecting to enroll at the right time could cause major financial and health-care headaches.

Chapter 8

REHAB AND LONG-TERM CARE

So far, we've mostly talked about Medicare's relationship with traditional medical care and services—things like doctor's visits, hospital stays, prescription medications, etc. As we age, though, the chances of us needing some form of enhanced care, like rehabilitation and long-term care services, increase exponentially. And these services can be incredibly expensive. Let's see how Medicare can help us out when we find ourselves faced with situations that reach beyond traditional medical services...

GET WELL SOON! COPING WITH INPATIENT REHABILITATION CARE

Sometimes, after surgery, an accident, or a serious illness, an extended period of inpatient rehabilitation therapy in a skilled-nursing facility is required in order to get us back on our feet and operating at our fullest capacity. If your physician certifies that you require medically necessary rehabilitative care, then you have some good news and some bad news. The bad news is that you have to spend some quality time at a rehab center, and you'll have to pay for some of it. The good news? Medicare is here to help!

In a rehab situation, Medicare Part A will cover...

- Rehabilitation services, including physical therapy, occupational therapy, and speech-language therapy
- A semi-private room
- Meals
- Nursing
- Drugs
- Other hospital services and supplies

Medicare Part A will NOT cover...

- Private nurses
- Telephones, televisions, or any other communications or entertainment services or devices
- Personal items, including hygiene and clothing articles

- A private room unless deemed medically necessary

HOW MUCH DOES IT COST?

When covering rehab services, Medicare Part A has some deductibles, each one of them applicable to a *single benefit period* (in other words, the deductibles apply from the date of your admittance to an inpatient facility to the sixtieth consecutive day after discharge. After that, if you are admitted again, a new benefit period begins).

In 2019, you will pay:

- Days one through sixty: A $1,364 total deductible (this is not owed if you were already admitted to a hospital within the same benefit period and satisfied the deductible there)

- Days sixty-one through ninety: $341.00 coinsurance each day
- Days ninety-one and beyond: $682.00 coinsurance for up to sixty days*
- After sixty days, you owe all costs

* This sixty-day period is known as your *lifetime reserve.* You have exactly sixty of them and they don't renew if you start a new benefit period. There is no way to get more. If you have any hospital stay over ninety days, your lifetime reserve is your last recourse before all costs are yours to cover. Nowadays, long hospital stays, in the traditional sense, are rare. If you're admitted to the hospital for an illness or injury, you'll probably be back home within a few days. Rehab, where long stays are still the norm, is the exception.

As you can see from the list of deductibles and coinsurance charges, above, the government is giving you a financial incentive to get in shape and go home. Doing otherwise can take a huge bite out of your wallet.

WHAT ROLE DOES MEDICARE PART B PLAY?

Medicare Part B still covers doctor's services, just like it normally would (see Chapter Two, "Medicare From A to D").

MIND THE THREE-DAY GAP

Before Medicare Part A will pay for any rehabilitation services, you must first be admitted to a hospital for at least three consecutive days. Less than that and Medicare will not pay. And here's a little tidbit that could trip you up: If you are in the hospital on an outpatient basis, and classified as *under observation,* you are not officially an *admitted patient*. Even if you spend the night (or the week), if you are classified as under observation, Medicare will not pay for follow-up rehab care. You must be officially classified as an admitted patient for three consecutive days for the rest of the machinery to kick in, and you are not admitted until the doctor says that you are ADMITTED. Be very aware of how long you have been admitted before moving on to rehab care. If you were admitted for less than three consecutive days (or not at all), and enroll in an inpatient rehab facility, you will pay for it. Literally.

THE LONG AND SHORT OF LONG-TERM CARE

Long-term care differs from rehab care in that it is designed to help those who are incapable of independently accomplishing two or more activities of daily living—like bathing, eating, toileting, dressing, standing from a sitting position—live their daily lives as comfortably and productively as possible in long-term care facilities (what we used to call nursing homes), or at home under the care of a skilled professional. As its name implies, those who find themselves in a long-term care situation are often in it for the long haul—in many cases for the rest of their lives. Needless to say, long-term care can be fabulously expensive.

BUT MEDICARE WILL PAY FOR IT, RIGHT?

Nope. Medicare will pay for skilled nursing care in a rehabilitation facility, where you are expected to eventually recover and go home, but it will not pay for care in an assisted-living facility (where your stay may be permanent), or for long-term care assistance at home.

WHAT ABOUT MEDIGAP INSURANCE?

Medigap plans are offered by private companies and may help pay for some long-term care costs—it's all up to the insurer. However, they routinely do not cover the costs of long-term care. Check with your provider to see what they may cover.

When it comes to long-term care, the bottom line is this: If you're concerned about it, look into an insurance policy that is designed specifically to cover long-term care needs. Unless you have a bank account with a long string of zeros at the end of it, your only other option will be to spend down your assets until you are classified as "low income," at which point Medicaid will take over and provide you with a bed in a Medicaid-certified facility. You'll be taken care of one way or another, but some ways are better than others.

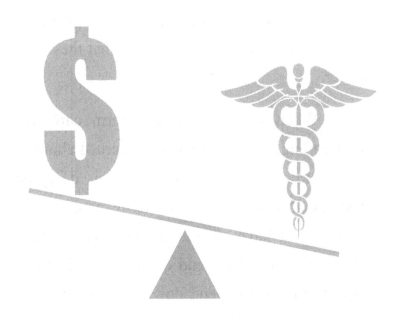

Chapter 9

THE FOUNTAIN OF YOUTH

Ah, the Fountain of Youth. The answer to all of our prayers. Take a drink and regain your youthful body without sacrificing your adult mind. Imagine that.

Sadly, that's not the Fountain of Youth that I'm talking about, but the one that I want to tell you about is still pretty cool. Here's how it works.

THE FORGETFUL EXECUTIVE RETIREE

Let's say that, after many years of faithful service, you retire from your company early, before the age of sixty-five, and receive a generous severance package which includes one hundred percent-paid COBRA health insurance. That's a pretty sweet deal, and not that uncommon.

Here's where the trouble arises. While you're sipping mai tais on the beach (or, more likely, shuttling the grandkids to soccer practice), you turn sixty-five. Big deal, right? You're already retired, you have your COBRA insurance, life is good. And who wants to celebrate turning sixty-five anyway? But while you're settled into your routine you may have forgotten something very important: When you turn sixty-five you MUST enroll in Medicare Parts B and D within eight months of your sixty-fifth birthday. Failure to do so will result in lifetime financial penalties for late enrollment *and* potentially a significant lapse in coverage while you wait for the open-enrollment period to come around. You could be without coverage for up to eight months. Not a good idea when you're over sixty-five.

"But wait!" you say. "I know I'm supposed to enroll in Medicare Parts B and D within eight months of my sixty-fifth birthday, and that failure to do so will result in lifetime financial penalties and possibly a significant lapse in coverage. But if I'm covered by an employer-paid COBRA plan, who cares? I'll just play dumb, ignore Medicare, and keep using COBRA to take care of my health-care needs."

I understand why you think you might get away with that, but there's one good reason why you won't: After your sixty-fifth birthday, Medicare becomes your *primary payer,* whether you're on COBRA or not. A routine surgery will put a stop to your scheme and open up a whole can of worms that, trust me, you don't want to deal with. Get enrolled and save yourself the trouble.

As I said earlier, though, most people just forget. It's understandable. You have a million things on your mind (I can't tell you how many times I've been told that retirement is busier than being employed). So what can you do? Do you have to accept the penalties or is there something you can do to avoid that hassle?

Maybe there is. Think outside of the box a little and you can drink from the Fountain of Youth! Remember from previous chapters (you read those, right?) that, when you come off of a employer's group plan, you have an open enrollment period in which you can enroll in Medicare Parts B and D without penalty or lapse of coverage. If you forgot to enroll in the midst of your COBRA plan, the solution is to turn back the clock and recreate your initial open-enrollment period.

Pulling this off will require some persuasive effort on your part, but it can be done. Approach your former employer, tell them what happened, and make sure they understand the importance of avoiding the late-enrollment penalties that you currently face (this is important; your previous employer may know very little about the rules of Medicare). Once you're sure they grasp the gravity of the situation, suggest the following solution: Rehire you and put you back on the group plan for thirty days. Like I said, you're going to have to be persuasive and talk them into it.

But it's worth it, and here's why: After your new thirty-day employment period, and you come off of your employer's group plan (for the second time), you will have a *new open enrollment period* and it will be just as if you have turned sixty-five all over again! Those penalties that were haunting you are washed away! Now go forth, my child, and ENROLL!

Chapter 10

SECTION 111 REPORTING

The rules of Medicare are written into US law and, as with any law, there are consequences when we don't follow it. In Chapter Four, "Medicare Secondary Payer," we looked at the various ways to determine whether Medicare or your private insurance carrier would be the primary or secondary carrier in various situations. It's essential that everyone involved in the Medicare process—employers, insurance companies, and individuals—pay close attention and know the rules (or at least have a reference— like this book!—to help keep things straight). Failure to do so could cost hundreds of thousands of dollars, which would be an unwelcome surprise to say the least.

Unfortunately, *failure to do so* is all too common. I get it. Medicare is the last thing that we want to think about. If you're like most people, when a health-care issue crosses your desk your priority is usually to take care of it as quickly as possible and make it disappear. You have more important things to do, right?

It's even worse if you're running a business. You're in business to make money, not to fiddle around with health care. The thing is, making a bad decision about Medicare enrollment could *cost your business money.* If you have employees on a company-provided health-insurance plan who are also enrolled in Medicare, it is in everyone's best interest to help those employees choose the right plan depending upon the number of employees at the company and any qualifying special conditions that the employee may have (see Chapter Four, "Medicare Secondary Payer," for more information).

THE IMPORTANCE OF COMPLIANCE

Section 111 compliance auditing refers to a mandatory auditing process in which the government gathers and examines information from insurers in order to confirm that individuals are properly enrolled in Medicare and that claims are being handled according to Medicare guidelines. If you are still covered by an employer health plan, and Medicare inappropriately paid a claim that they should not have paid on your or your spouse's behalf, the government may seek reimbursement from your employer, and the amounts could run into the hundreds of thousands of dollars. That's bad enough if you're the employee; if you're the employer you could be looking at a serious hit to your bottom line.

Improper claims cost employers thousands of dollars in premiums, insurance companies hundreds of thousands to millions of dollars in payments, and our government millions to billions of dollars in payments. It adds up, and finding out that you have to make up for an error that could have been easily prevented can really ruin your day.

Here's an example of how things could go wrong: Using the categories in Chapter Four ("Medicare Secondary Payer"), let's say that you are in Category 2 (Your company offers a health plan and has twenty or more employees). In this case, Medicare would be the *secondary* payer. If the claim is filed improperly, and Medicare pays first (instead of the insurance company), your employer is likely to receive a bill for reimbursement.

Here's another, more complex, example: You may recall that if a spouse of an employee who is covered on an employer-sponsored group plan through a company that has a hundred or more employees (including part-time and seasonal staff), becomes disabled, and applies for Social Security disability income, Medicare is the *secondary* payer and should not pay any claims. The employer's insurance company should pay that claim, not Medicare. If Medicare is erroneously billed, and the error is discovered through Section 111 auditing, Medicare *can,* probably *will,* and definitely *have* come back to employers for those monies. Once again, we are talking about amounts that are potentially in the hundreds of thousands of dollars. Ouch.

On the flip side, if the employer's group has two to ninety-nine employees, Medicare is the *primary* payer and *should* pay this claim, *not* the insurance company. Smaller companies typically don't have the robust HR support that larger companies have and are therefore more likely to make these kinds of errors. While insurance companies generally can't come back and demand reimbursement the way that the government can, compliance errors and improper billing cost insurers millions of dollars in claims that Medicare should be paying which, in turn, drives up insurance costs for *everyone*.

It is incumbent upon all of us—the government, insurance companies, our employers, and ourselves—to ensure that everyone pays attention and that the rules are followed. It's the only way to guarantee that we receive the care to which we're entitled without the risk of unpleasant surprises and crippling financial consequences.

CONCLUSION: MAKING MEDICARE WORK TODAY, TOMORROW, AND INTO THE FUTURE

Every generation faces its own challenges, adapts to meet them, and then passes along the tools to the next generation. Sometimes those tools become rusty and obsolete and have to be repaired, sharpened, or even replaced with something entirely different. The US Constitution addresses the challenges of a largely agrarian republic of the 1780s, not a highly urbanized, post-industrial twenty-first century society. The Founding Fathers' crowning achievement is still with us because it has changed with the times.

In 1963, when President Lyndon Johnson signed Medicare into law, the average American lived to the very young age of seventy. Now, in 2019, the average female, if she reaches age sixty-five, can expect to live to ninety-three, and a male who attains age sixty-five will live to approximately age eighty-eight. Our children, who are now aged thirty to thirty-five, may expect to live to the ripe old age of one hundred, if not longer. Where will this all end? Will life spans continue to expand? Will we have an ever-growing senior population? The answer is simple: We may never know. We certainly don't know now. And that's why we must look at making some changes. The architects of Medicare couldn't see the future. Their crowning achievement was not designed to cope with the challenges of the twenty-first century.

And there have been changes—Medicare Parts C and D weren't part of the original plan—but the core issue of an aging population that outstrips Medicare's capabilities has yet to be addressed. Our children's and grandchildren's financial futures depends upon us. We have to act, with purpose and vision, to bring this midcentury beast into the twenty-first century.

The most fundamental change, the one modification that is essential to the very survival of the system, is to raise the Medicare eligibility age from sixty-five to seventy. We're all living longer, we're all working longer, but our healthcare system assumes that it's 1966 and we still have seventy-year life expectancies. Baby Boomers are aging into Medicare at the torrid pace of a thousand a day, and close to twenty percent of the Boomers' parents are still alive, adding fuel to the fire and are bleeding our nation's financial nest egg. By the year 2026, one-third of our population will be sixty-five or older. And our workforce is aging. Over thirty million Americans are still working full-time between ages sixty-five and seventy-eight. Our caregivers need a financial future. We must all work together as a team to slow the bleeding. We can't stop the bleeding, that's virtually impossible, but if we put our heads together we can come up with a mutually agreeable solution. We don't really have a choice.

Medicare for All is an idea that is on a lot of people's minds as the country lurches into the 2020 presidential-election season. *Medicare for All* proposes a national healthcare solution that pays for the healthcare of citizens who are below the age of sixty-five, almost like socialized medicine in Europe. That would be a sweeping, holistic change with far-reaching consequences that would reach into every corner of our economy and our society. Whether this would be good or bad in the long run I don't know, but it would certainly be disruptive and we'd all endure some pain before the system got up and running at full throttle. Any number of changes could be made to deal with our non-senior population, but my specialty is seniors and here's how I think the system could be reformed so that we can care for our aging population without draining our national bank account.

As mentioned earlier, we must change Medicare eligibility to age seventy, not sixty-five. Those who are between sixty-five and the new eligibility age of seventy will be enrolled in a brand-new preliminary healthcare program that pays fifty percent of all healthcare services. This offers an olive branch to those who are already nearly sixty-five when the change takes effect, and eases participants into the full Medicare system into which they will now be enrolled at age seventy.

It may not seem like a huge change, but the payoff would be enormous. One thousand Americans reach age sixty-five, and age into Medicare, every day. Multiply that by 365 days and, over the next six years (through 2026) over 2.2 million Americans will have aged into Medicare. The average cost to fund (claims, healthcare services, etc.) a Medicare beneficiary in 2019 is close to $10,000 per month. You do the math! Raising the Medicare age to seventy will save trillions of dollars, the equivalent of balancing the budget for two sitting presidents! Just a thought! Somebody has to think about what we can do to preserve the financial backbone of our children and grandchildren. The future of our youth depends on it. Our forefathers had no idea that their country would grow to be as large as 350 million people, and that we would, on average, live three times longer than they could have imagined. I know President Johnson didn't! Their intensions were good. Ours must be better (and smarter)! And whatever changes are made, the government must do a better job of communicating both the rules and the opportunities of Medicare to the American public. It often seems as if Medicare is a mystery, its secrets and intricacies known only to a small group of experts. It shouldn't be that way. Medicare must be brought fully and robustly into the 21st century, and it must be so crystal-clear that the average American can comprehend it with ease and implement it with confidence.

We can do it. We put men on the moon and launched spacecraft that travel beyond our solar system. We have a postal service that delivers mail to every single address in this country six days a week. Our massive military operation fields forces in every corner of the globe. Those are challenges. Those are hard. Designing a healthcare system that takes care of our parents and grandparents without breaking the bank seems pretty easy by comparison. We just have to summon the will to make it a reality. We can do it.

Our society and the marketplace do not have a Healthcare Cost Crisis. We do not even have a Healthcare Crisis. We have a Health Crisis. As soon as we all understand this, and the real issues, then, and only then, will we be able to create solutions, and achieve profound financial strides, as we navigate through the 21st Century.

Rick Solofsky

APPENDIX 1: COVID-19

Nothing ever goes as planned. I poured my soul into this book, spent countless nights slaving away over a hot keyboard, published it, everybody said *Wow, great book, Rick,* and then COVID-19 came along and threw a rock right through my window.

Now I am not trying to make light of a deadly disease, or imply that the minor inconvenience of having to revise this book in any way compares to the hardships that some of us have had to endure—far from it—but I do try to keep a sense of humor about it. But revise this book I must, so here we go:

SO WHAT'S WITH COVID-19?

First of all—and this is important—none of the fundamental information in this book is changed by COVID-19. Everything still works just as I said it would, there's just a temporary adjustment for those who were impacted during a specific span of time. And you can rest easy because it's pretty simple:

If your initial enrollment window for Medicare Part A or Part B was between March 17th and June 17th, 2020, and you missed it due to government office closures or other lack of access caused by COVID-19, your enrollment window is extended to September 17th, 2020 with no late-enrollment penalties.

Likewise, if you missed a Medicare Part D or Medicare Advantage (Part C) enrollment that should have been made between March 1st and June 30st, 2020 (note that this is a different span of dates than was used for Parts A and B) due to COVID-19 closures, you will also be able to enroll at a later date.

COVID-19 issues are still in flux and there is no guarantee that what you just read is still current. Here are links and QR codes (scan them with your phone's bar-code reader) that, as of the time of this writing, will take you to up-to-date information straight from the government, including enrollment instructions.

FOR MEDICARE PARTS A AND B

Link: https://go.cms.gov/2TWus0Y

QR code:

FOR MEDICARE PART C

Link: https://go.cms.gov/3cqJZwa

QR code:

FOR MEDICARE PART D

Link: https://go.cms.gov/3ewNov0

QR code:

APPENDIX 2: SECTION 105

Wouldn't it be awesome if your employer could pay your Medicare premiums? Yes, it would be. Unfortunately, they are legally barred from doing so. However, as is often the case, there is a creative way around this issue and it's pretty cool.

WHAT DO YOU WANT FIRST,
THE GOOD NEWS OR THE BAD NEWS?

Let's start with the bad news: No matter what, you still have to pay your premiums. That doesn't change; there's no way of getting out of it. But here's the good news: A Section 105 plan allows an employer to make tax-free contributions to a fund that can be used to reimburse employees for a number of medical expenses, including vision and dental care, orthodontia, physician and lab fees, chiropractic care, psychiatric care, prescription costs, and (drum roll please) *Medicare premiums!* In other words, you still have to pay your premiums, but your employer, through a Section 105 plan, could reimburse you.

This is a fantastic program, especially for businesses with older workforces, and a great, relatively low-cost employee benefit that many employers know nothing about. If you're an employer, there are several types of Section 105 plans available, some of which may even provide significant tax savings for your bottom line, but how the plan works depends upon how your business is classified. Check with your tax advisor to make sure you pick the plan that works best for you, your business, and your employees, but above all, *look into it.* You'll reap the benefits, and your employees will thank you every time they pay a premium.

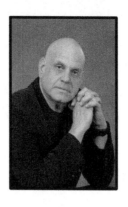

Rick Solofsky, a 1979 graduate of West Chester State University, has over thirty years of experience as a health-care broker and high-level consultant with a specialty in Medicare and the interpretation of "Medicare Secondary Payer Law" and how it applies to the group insurance culture. Today, Solofsky Financial Group administers over 150 group health-care accounts in Pennsylvania and New Jersey, in addition to over 300 individuals, and Medicare-supplement policies for more than 400 individuals. Rick frequently educates other brokers, CPAs, and attorneys about changes in the Medicare/health-insurance landscape. A regular contributor to many financial talk shows, Rick credits his dual major—Health/Physical Education *and* Psychology— with helping him better understand the "Big Picture" of the role of health insurance in American life.

Get in touch—Rick is here to help!

Phone/Text: 215-432-7425

Email: Rick@SolofskyFG.com

Solofsky Financial Group on the web: www.SolofskyFG.com

122

Made in the USA
Middletown, DE
11 February 2021

33567616R00076